W0042340

T E X T

THE R_f APEUTICS

Judy McIntosh

Text Therapeutics

Judy McIntosh

ISBN 978-0-7923-6901-1   ISBN 978-94-010-0773-3 (eBook)
DOI 10.1007/978-94-010-0773-3

Printed on acid-free paper

All Rights Reserved
© 2001 Springer Science+Business Media New York
Originally published by Kluwer Academic Publishers in 2001

Notice of Rights

All rights reserved. No part of this book may be reproduced, stored in a retrieval system or transmitted in any form by any means, electronic, mechanical, photocopying, recording, or otherwise, without prior written permission from the author/publisher.

Notice of Liability

The examples in this book are distributed as English text references only and not as official medical science references or as official medical treatment protocols or as official medical trial results. The information in this book is distributed on an 'As is' basis, and the author/publisher shall be without warranty or liability to any person or entity.

Dedication

To my dear friend, Anastasia Skandalis, MD, who throughout the writing of this book was an unfailing source of invaluable expertise, suggestions and encouragement. I am truly grateful.

Acknowledgements

In the preparation of this book, the following excellent references were consulted:

Collins Cobuild English Language Dictionary. Collins Birmingham University International Database. J. Sinclair, P. Hanks, G. Fox, R. Moon, P. Stock, editors. London: William Collins Sons & Co Ltd, 1988.

Quirk, R. and Greenbaum, S. *A University Grammar of English*. Harlow: Longman, 1984.

Swan, M. *Practical English Usage*. Oxford: Oxford University Press, 1995.

Special Thanks

To Sue Garnett, MA, for her scholarly insight and recommendations, and to Jo Harding, who with a keen eye proof-read the manuscript.

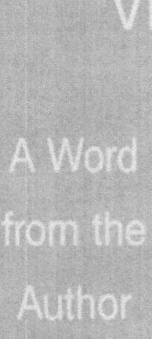

A Word
from the
Author

By way of **introduction**, this book was written specifically for medical science professionals whose mother tongue is *not* English. Writing top-level papers for medical journals of international repute and oral presentations for worldwide medical congresses demands a certain linguistic dexterity. Thinking in one's own language and translating directly into English often results in stilted text fraught with word order problems and grammatical errors.

The **objective** of *Text Therapeutics* is to assist all medical science non-native speakers in the task of writing professional research documents in English.

With regard to **materials and methods**, *Text Therapeutics* provides a series of 'error extracts' coupled with corrected text and a follow-the-formula analysis with convenient categorized side-headings. Errors and text problems are precisely pinpointed and easily understood. Other sections of *Text Therapeutics* are indicated in the 'Table of Contents' on the next page.

The **results** are now in the form of the book you are holding in your hand.

In **conclusion**, it is my hope that *Text Therapeutics* proves to be a valuable and practical English language reference tool. Further books are scheduled at a future date.
Thank you for taking the time to read this book and I extend my sincere wishes for every success in the publication and/or presentation of your clinical or laboratory research.

Judy McIntosh
Athens,
November, 2000

VII

Table
of
Contents

Correct text in the 'error extract' is printed **like this.** Grey print indicates errors or text that can be improved: these areas are classed according to one or more of the side-heading categories. A √ in the explanations is the symbol for correct text, but the suggested usage is preferable.

Corrected text is printed next to 'text therapeutics' in bold like this.

A V Ø I D   • inadvisable ITEMS

Grammar Glimpse   • grammatical APPLICATIONS

in *brief*   • concise DATA

insight   • advanced language TOOLS

notes   • your own MEDICAL excerpts

prepositions   • prepositional GUIDELINES

Specify   • clarifying the text PICTURE

verb ease   • simplified verb RESOLUTIONS

→
WORD ORDER   • effective syntactical FORMULAS
←

Word - *Wise*   • vocabulary IMPROVEMENT

c r o s s   REFERENCES   • grammar glimpse = *G*, specify = S, verb ease = v, word order = *W* + related pages

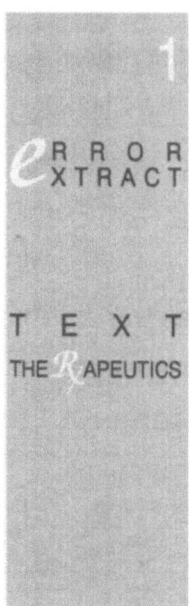

ERROR EXTRACT

These data broaden the currently available knowledge about the progression of the disease and may allow to define distinct factors of prognostic relevance.

TEXT

THE APEUTICS

These data broaden the currently available knowledge **related to disease progression** and **may allow a definition** of (**may allow us to define**) distinct factors of prognostic relevance.

in *brief*

• disease progression = the progression of the disease √

verb ease

• allow + noun = allow + (a) definition (of distinct factors)

• allow + somebody + to do something = allow + us + to define (distinct factors)

Word - *Wise*

• related to = regarding = about √

notes

•

cross REFERENCES

• v 3.6.48.   •

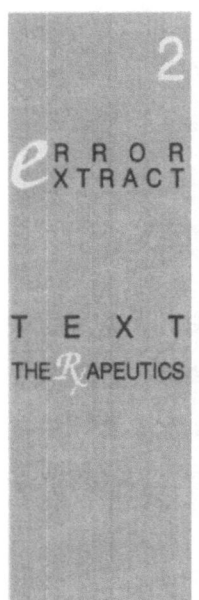

2

ERROR EXTRACT

During the years 1997 to 2000 **a total of 37 autologous stem cell transplants** have been performed **at our institution** for lymphoproliferative diseases.

TEXT

THERAPEUTICS

In total, 37 autologous stem cell transplants for lymphoproliferative diseases **were performed** at our institution **from June 1997 to June 2000**.

verb ease

• simple past tense > completed action > specific time in the past = were performed + from June 1997 to June 2000

WORD ORDER

• place related words and phrases next to each other = subject + modifier = stem cell transplants + for lymphoproliferative diseases

Specify

• state month and year = from June 1997 to June 2000

notes

•

c r o s s
REFERENCES

• v 9.10.16.20.22.26.28. • *W* 18.• S 22.   •

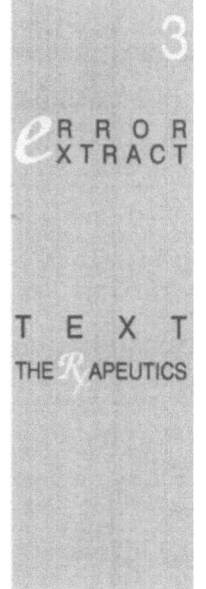

3

ERROR
EXTRACT

The small number in this series doesn't allow to draw any firm conclusions: however we think that both treatment modalities achieve similar results and the quality of life is better in the former group of patients.

T E X T
THE APEUTICS

The small number in this series **does not allow us to draw** any firm conclusions. However, **in our opinion**, **although** both treatment modalities achieve similar results, the quality of life is better in the former group of patients.

A V Ø I D

- contractions should not be used in professional publications: does not = doesn't √

verb ease

- allow + somebody + to do something = allow + us + to draw (any firm conclusions)

insight

- although + statement + second unexpected statement = although + both treatment modalities achieve similar results, + [rather unexpectedly] the quality of life is better in the former group of patients

Word - *Wise*

- in our opinion = we think √

notes

-

cross
REFERENCES

- v 1.6.48.   •

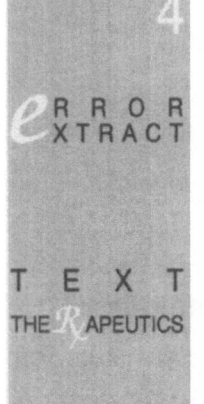

4

ERROR EXTRACT

.So far we could not find any clinical variables that can predict the group of patients at a higher risk of failure.

TEXT

THE ℛ APEUTICS

So far we **have not been able to find** any clinical variables that can **determine** the group of patients at a **higher failure risk**.

verb ease

- present perfect tense > an action that started in the past and which is ongoing in the present = so far + present perfect tense = so far + we have not been able to find

Word - *Wise*

- determine = ascertain = discover ≠ predict

in *brief*

- a higher failure risk = a higher risk of failure √

notes

-

c r o s s
REFERENCES

- v 8.11.12.17.23.24.25.26.34.   •

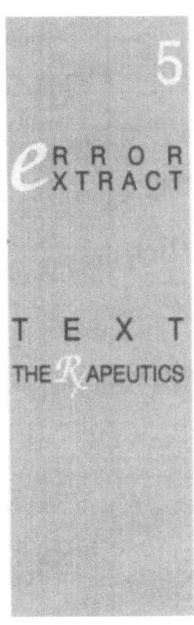

5 Further investigations are undergoing.

T E X T

THE RAPEUTICS

Further investigations **are underway**.

verb ease

- present continuous tense > an action which is happening now = are undergoing = are being subjected to: e.g. The patients are undergoing surgery at this moment.

Word - *Wise*

- investigations are underway = activities that are now taking place

notes

-

cross
REFERENCES

- v 15.18.

-

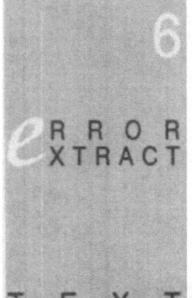

6

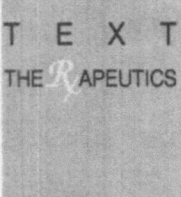

ERROR EXTRACT

In conclusion, **this series** does not permit to conclude definitely to **the potential value of such an approach.**

TEXT

THE APEUTICS

In summary, this series **does not permit (us to form) a definite conclusion as to (regarding)** the potential value of such an approach.

AVØID
- repetitive usage: in summary = in conclusion √; 'in summary' is used here to avoid the use of 'conclusion' and 'conclude' in the same sentence

Word - *Wise*
- as to = regarding = related to

verb ease
- permit = allow + somebody + to do something = permit + us + to form (a definite conclusion)

- permit = allow + noun = permit + (a definite) conclusion

Grammar Glimpse
- adjective + noun = (a) definite + conclusion

cross REFERENCES
- v 1.3.48. • *G* 9.10.22.

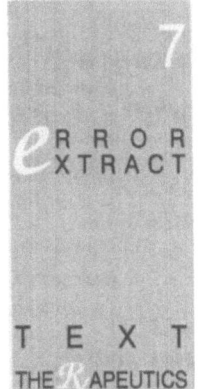

ERROR
EXTRACT

Shortened progression-free survival (PFS) and survival was associated with performance status which was impaired, **spleen involvement, anaemia and a low serum albumin level.**

TEXT
THE *R* APEUTICS

Shortened progression-free survival (PFS) and survival **were associated** with **impaired performance status**, spleen involvement, anaemia and a low serum albumin level.

Grammar Glimpse

- plural subject + plural verb = progression-free survival and survival + were associated

in *brief*

- impaired performance status = performance status which was impaired √

notes

-

cross
REFERENCE

- *G* 41.

-

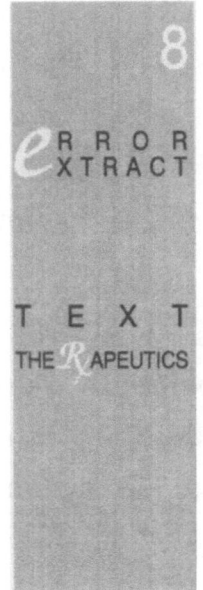

8

Regularly in these patients ultrasonography is used to assess the appearance of early disease symptoms but its role is not yet clearly defined.

T E X T

THE *R* APEUTICS

In these patients, ultrasonography is **regularly** used to assess the appearance of early disease symptoms but its role **has not yet been** clearly **defined** (**has not been** clearly **defined yet**).

WORD ORDER

- adverbs of frequency are usually placed between two-part verbs = is + regularly + used

verb ease

- present perfect tense > an action that started in the past and which up to now has not been accomplished = not yet + present perfect tense = has not yet been (clearly) defined = has not been (clearly) defined yet

notes

•

c r o s s
REFERENCES

• v 4.11.12.17.23.24.25.26.34. • *W* 10.25.37.   •

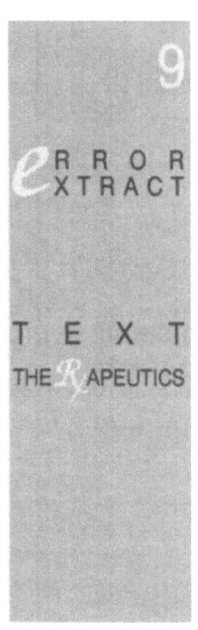

9

e R R O R
X T R A C T

Six-years results have been published in 1998.

T E X T

THE _Rx_ APEUTICS

Six-**year** results **were published** in 1998.

Grammar Glimpse

- years = plural noun; cardinal number + plural noun used as an adjective (the 's' is dropped) + noun = six + year + results = six-year results

verb ease

- simple past tense > completed action > specific time in the past = were published + in 1998

notes

-

c r o s s
REFERENCES

- _G_ 6.10.22. • v 2.10.16.20.22.26.28.
•

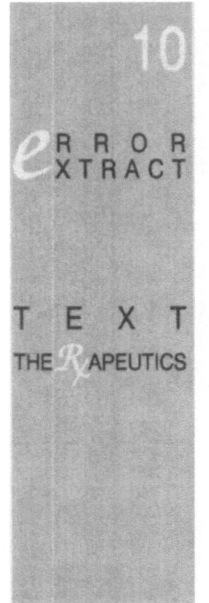

10

e R R O R
X T R A C T

To February 2000, **320 patients** have been accrued, 250 being evaluated for clinic features.

T E X T
THE ℞APEUTICS

Up to February 2000, 320 patients were accrued, 250 of whom were clinically evaluated (were evaluated clinically).

prepositions

• up to = up until > an action or situation which stops at the time mentioned = up to + February 2000

verb ease

• simple past tense > completed action = were accrued + February 2000

in *brief*

• 250 of whom were clinically evaluated = 250 of whom were evaluated for clinical features √

*G*rammar *G*limpse

• adjective + noun = clinical + features

→
WORD ORDER
←

• adverbs of manner (> 'how' something is done) ending in 'ly' are usually placed between or after two-part verbs = were + clinically + evaluated = were + evaluated + clinically

c r o s s
REFERENCES

• v 2.9.16.20.22.26.28. • *G* 6.9.22. • *W* 8.25.37. •

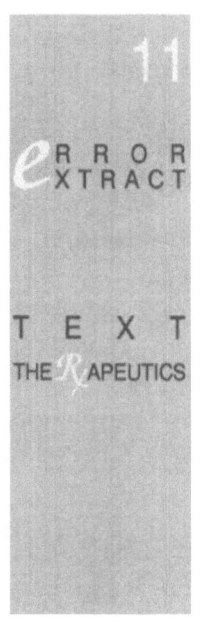

11

*e*RROR
XTRACT

To date, only 12/150 patients presented with progressive disease or relapse.

T E X T
THE *R* APEUTICS

To date, only 12/150 patients **have presented** with progressive disease or relapse.

verb ease

- present perfect tense > an action that started in the past and which continues in the present = to date = so far + present perfect tense = to date + (12/150 patients) have presented

notes

-

c r o s s
REFERENCES

- v 4.8.12.17.23.24.25.26.34.

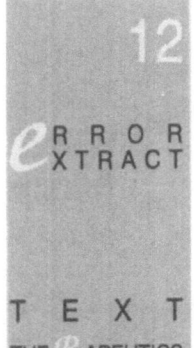

ERROR
EXTRACT

Up to now, the long-term immunosuppressive effect and its consequences are not evaluated nor is remission duration.

TEXT
THE ℞APEUTICS

Up to now, the long-term immunosuppressive effect and its consequences **have not been evaluated** nor **has** remission duration.

verb ease

- present perfect tense > an action that started in the past and which is ongoing in the present = up to now = so far = to date + present perfect tense = up to now + (the immunosuppressive effect and its consequences) + have not been evaluated + (nor) has (= has remission duration been evaluated)

notes

-

cross
REFERENCES

- v 4.8.11.17.23.24.25.26.34.   •

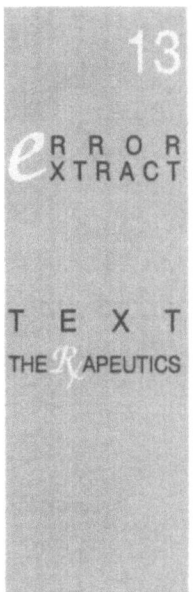

13

The intensification of regimens for patients with risk factors allowed to improve the treatment outcome.

ERROR
EXTRACT

TEXT

THE RAPEUTICS

Regimen intensification for **risk factor patients resulted in an improvement** in treatment outcome.

in *brief*

- regimen intensification = intensification of regimens √

- risk factor patients = patients with risk factors √

Word - *Wise*

- allowed = permitted ≠ resulted in

- resulted in = brought about a certain outcome = resulted in + an improvement

notes

-

c r o s s
REFERENCES

-

-

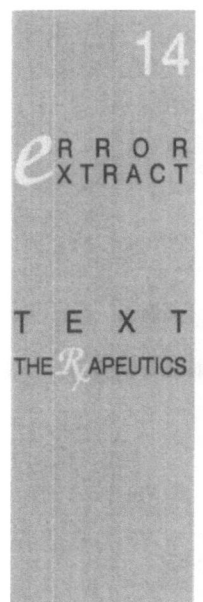

14

However, this combination therapy is difficult to be performed because of the related bone marrow toxicity.

T E X T
THE *R* APEUTICS

However, because of the related bone marrow toxicity, this combination therapy is difficult **to administer**.

Word - *Wise*

- therapy is administered ≠ performed: e.g. Combination therapy was administered. Surgery was performed.

verb ease

- to administer + something (+ to somebody) = to administer + this combination therapy (+ to patients) = this combination therapy is difficult to administer (to patients)

notes

-

c r o s s
REFERENCES

-

-

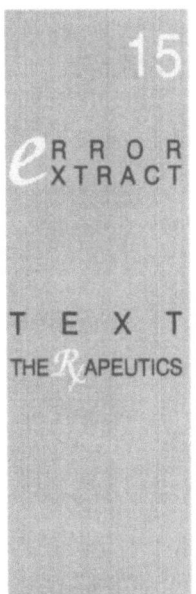

15

*e*RROR
XTRACT

The patient must be fasting for 3-4 hours before the examination.

TEXT

THE *R*APEUTICS

The patient **must fast** for 3-4 hours before the examination.

verb ease

- present continuous tense > an action which is happening at this moment: e.g. The patient is fasting now.

- the patient must be fasting = I assume that the patient is fasting now (because the doctor told him/her to fast for 3-4 hours before the examination).

- must + bare infinitive = the patient + must + fast = The patient is obliged to fast (for 3-4 hours before the examination).

notes

-

cross
REFERENCES

- v 5.18.

-

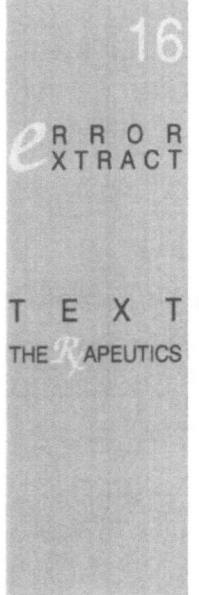

16

*e*R R O R
XTRACT

Following this procedure, the material had
been **cytologically** evaluated.

T E X T
THE *R* APEUTICS

Following this procedure, the material **was**
cytologically **evaluated**.

verb ease

- simple past tense > completed action =
  was cytologically evaluated (following this
  procedure)

- past perfect tense > an action which took
  place before another action which is
  mentioned > usually the earlier action in
  the past = past perfect tense + later action
  in the past = simple past tense = following
  this procedure = (after this procedure had
  been performed) + the material was
  evaluated; see 'insight' below:

insight

- when the two past actions take place within close time proximity, sometimes the
  simple past tense is used for both = the
  procedure was performed + the material
  was evaluated

c r o s s
REFERENCES

- v 2.9.10.20.22.26.28.   •

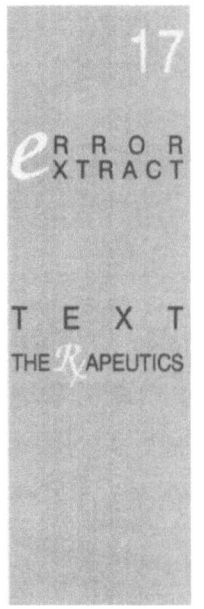

17

e R R O R
X T R A C T

Thus far, no successful treatment modality
is established.

T E X T

THE *R* APEUTICS

Thus far, no successful treatment modality
has been established.

verb ease

• present perfect tense > an action which
began in the past and is ongoing now =
thus far = so far = to date = up to now +
present perfect tense = thus far (no
successful treatment modality) + has
been established

notes

•

c r o s s
REFERENCES

• v 4.8.11.12.23.24.25.26.34.   •

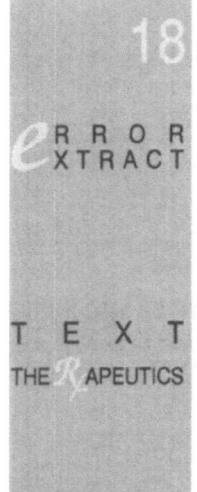

ERROR
EXTRACT

In a multi-centre randomised study we currently evaluate whether or not this treatment modality is useful in high risk patients in preventing infections **namely those mediated by the herpes virus.**

TEXT
THERAPEUTICS

In a multi-centre randomised study **of high risk patients, we are** currently **evaluating the usefulness** of this treatment modality **in preventing infections,** namely those mediated by the herpes virus.

verb ease

- present continuous tense > an action which is happening now or in the general present = currently + present continuous tense = we are currently evaluating

- evaluate + noun = evaluating + the usefulness (of this treatment)

in *brief*

- evaluating the usefulness of this treatment modality = evaluating whether or not this treatment modality is useful √

Word Order

- noun + modifier = (a multi-centre randomised) study + of high risk patients

- the usefulness of this treatment modality + in preventing infections

c r o s s
REFERENCES

- v. 5.15. • W 2.   •

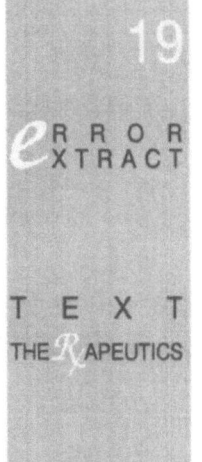

19

e R R O R
X T R A C T

Further investigations are needed for searching a new effective chemotherapy.

T E X T
THE *R*APEUTICS

In the search for a new effective chemotherapy **regimen**, further investigations are **required**.

prepositions

- in the search for + noun = in the search for + (a new effective chemotherapy) regimen

- for + 'ing' > used when something mentioned requires explaining or justifying: e.g. There are serious reasons for searching for a new effective regimen.

Specify

- state what = chemotherapy + regimen

Word - *Wise*

- required = needed √

notes

-

c r o s s
REFERENCES

- S 34.38.49.

-

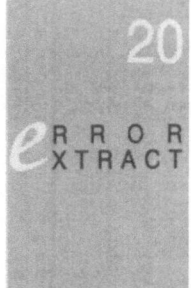

20

A significant improvement in the quality of life is observed after **four** week **treatment**.

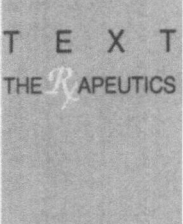

TEXT
THE *R* APEUTICS

A significant improvement in the quality of life **was observed following** four **weeks of** treatment.

verb ease
- simple past tense > completed action = was observed + following four weeks of treatment

Word - *Wise*
- following = after √

*G*rammar *G*limpse
- plural number + plural noun = four + weeks

notes
-

cross REFERENCES
- v 2.9.10.16.22.26.28. • *G* 45. •

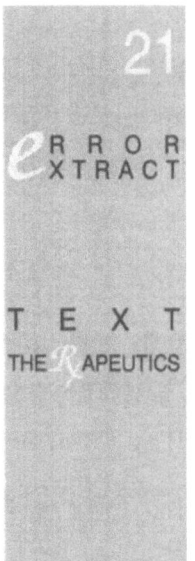

21

It is also unknown the exact percentage of benign apparently gastric ulcers that are instead ulcerated malignant lesions.

T E X T

THE ℛ APEUTICS

The exact percentage of **apparently** benign gastric ulcers that are, **in reality**, ulcerated malignant lesions, is also unknown.

Grammar Glimpse

- it = the exact percentage; use either as the subject, but not both = the exact percentage + is also unknown

- adverb + adjectives + noun = apparently + benign + gastric + ulcers

insight

- instead = adverb + verb > to indicate that something else is done in place of another action that is mentioned: e.g. The surgeon intended to start his vacation but instead he found himself performing major surgery.

- instead of = as opposed to + 'ing': e.g. Instead of starting his vacation the surgeon found himself performing major surgery.

c r o s s
REFERENCES

- G 34.36.   •

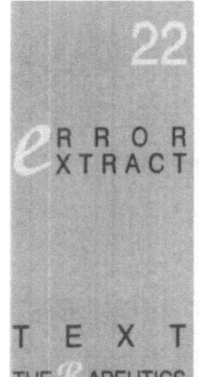

eRROR
XTRACT

In a multi-centre protocol from 1990 to 1995, 89 patients (53 men, 36 women) with Stage III-IV intermediate and high grade non-Hodgkin's lymphoma (NHL) have been treated.

TEXT
THE RAPEUTICS

In a multi-centre protocol from **January** 1990 to **December** 1995, 89 patients (53 **male**, 36 **female**) with Stage III-IV intermediate and high grade non-Hodgkin's lymphoma (NHL) **were treated**.

Specify

- state exact dates: from January 1990 to December 1995

Grammar Glimpse

- adjective + noun = 89 patients (53 male, 36 female patients)

verb ease

- simple past tense > completed action > specific time in the past (January 1990 to December 1995) = were treated

notes

-

cross
REFERENCES

- S 2. *G* 6.9.10. • v 2.9.10.16.20.26.28. •

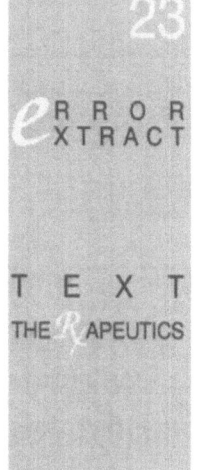

23

eRROR
XTRACT

According to other authors, no significant differences are seen between complete remission (CR), survival and disease-free survival cases.

T E X T
THE *R* APEUTICS

According to other authors, no significant differences **have been seen among** complete remission (CR), survival and disease-free survival cases.

verb ease

- present perfect tense > an action which started in the past and which continues in the present; although not directly stated, the underlying meaning is: according to what other authors have written to date; to date + present perfect tense = to date (no significant differences) + have been seen

*G*rammar
limpse

- between > two persons, places, objects

- among > more than two persons, places, objects = among complete remission (CR), survival and disease-free survival cases

cross
REFERENCES

- v 4.8.11.12.17.24.25.26.34.   •

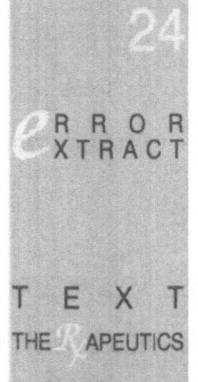

eRROR
XTRACT

TEXT

THE *R* APEUTICS

The prognostic role in distinguishing histology of a low grade from histology of a high grade is not yet **clearly** outlined **and** requires further investigation.

The prognostic role in distinguishing **low-grade histology from high-grade histology has not yet been** clearly **outlined (has not been** clearly **outlined yet)** and requires further investigation.

in *brief*

- low-grade histology = histology of a low grade √; high-grade histology = histology of a high grade √

verb ease

- present perfect tense > an action that started in the past and which up to now has not been accomplished = not yet + present perfect tense = has not yet been (clearly) outlined = has not been (clearly) outlined yet

notes

-

c r o s s
REFERENCES

- v 4.8.11.12.17.23.25.26.34.

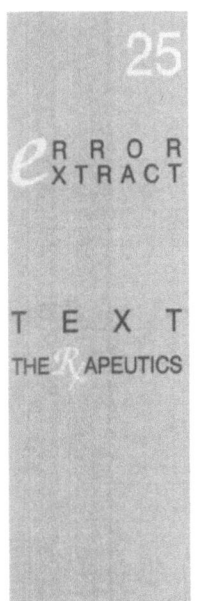

*e*RROR XTRACT

T E X T
THE*R*APEUTICS

At our iinstitution, from Sept. 2000, there is an ongıoing study in which patients affected with acivanced-stage disease randomly are allocatœd to receive 6 therapy cycles.

At our institution, **since Sept. 2000**, there **has been** an ongoing study in which **advanced-stage disease patients are randomly allocated (are allocated randomly)** to receive 6 therapy cycles.

verb ease

- since > often indicates an event or occurrence which started at a past time mentioned (Sept. 2000) and which continues in the present time = since + present perfect tense = since + Sept. 2000 + there has been

in *brief*

- advanced-stage disease patients = patients affected with advanced-stage disease √

WORD ORDER

- adverbs of manner (> 'how' something is done) ending in 'ly' are usually placed between or after two-part verbs = are + randomly + allocated = are + allocated + randomly

c r o s s
REFERENCES

- v 4.8.11.12.17.23.24.26.34. • *W* 8.10.37.   •

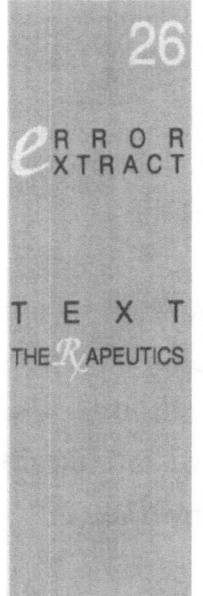

26

*e*RROR
XTRACT

Numerous studies ~~were carried out~~ in recent years.

T E X T

THE *R*APEUTICS

Numerous studies **have been carried out** in recent years.

verb ease

- in recent years = recently + present perfect tense when referring to a *time period* before or until now = in recent years (numerous studies) + present perfect tense = have been carried out

- recently > sometimes refers to a *point in time* when an action or occurrence took place = recently + simple past tense: e.g. She was recently appointed as head of the Bone Marrow Transplantation Unit.

notes

-

cross
REFERENCES

- v 4.8.11.12.17.23.24.25.34. • 2.9.10.16.20.22.28.•

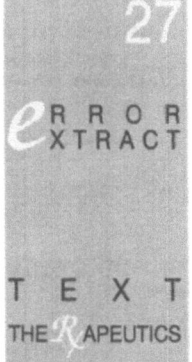

27

ERROR EXTRACT

Only a low percentage of patients need in acute ulcer bleeding surgical intervention.

T E X T
THE *R* APEUTICS

Only a low percentage of patients **with acute ulcer bleeding requires** surgical intervention.

*G*rammar *G*limpse

- singular subject + singular verb = only a low percentage (of patients) + requires

Word - *Wise*

- requires = needs √

prepositions

- with > a physical characteristic or characteristics = with acute ulcer bleeding = patients who have acute ulcer bleeding

*W*ORD *O*RDER

- subject + modifier + verb = a low percentage of patients + with acute ulcer bleeding + requires

notes

-

c r o s s
REFERENCES

- *G* 40.50. • *W* 30.33.36.37.47.48.51. •

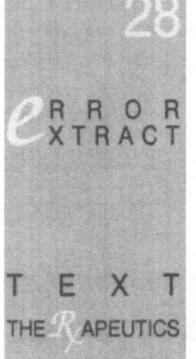

e R R O R
X T R A C T

92 patients have been accrued and 86 met the criteria to be included in the study.

T E X T
THE *R* APEUTICS

Of the 92 patients **accrued**, 86 met **the inclusion criteria** of the study.

prepositions

- of the = out of the > something that happens to one or several persons who are selected from a larger group = of the + 92 patients + 86 (met the inclusion criteria)

A V Ø I D

- 92 = ninety-two: medical journals usually specify that numbers at the beginning of the sentence should be written in full

verb ease

- simple past tense > completed action = (of the 92 patients) accrued + (86) met

in *brief*

- the inclusion criteria = the criteria to be included √

c r o s s
REFERENCES

- v 2.9.10.16.20.22.26.

•

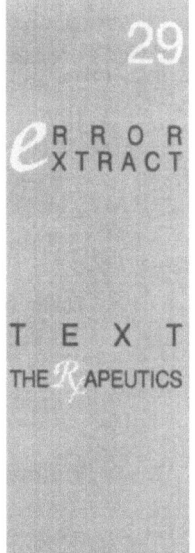

ERROR EXTRACT

We conclude that there is a need for revision of existing indices **and recommend** that an item-bias detection strategy is included as an early and essential step in the development of new indices.

TEXT

THE *R* APEUTICS

We conclude that existing indices **require revision** and recommend that an item-bias detection strategy **be** included as an early and essential step in the development of new indices.

in *brief*

- existing indices require revision = there is a need for revision of existing indices √

insight

- recommend that + noun + bare infinitive = recommend that + (an item-bias detection) strategy + be (included): e.g. The physician recommended that the patient rest.

notes

-

cross REFERENCES

-

-

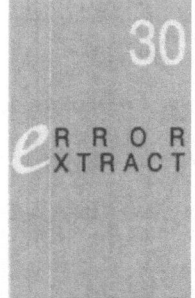

eRROR
XTRACT

The preliminary results show how rare a condition is ulcerative colitis.

TEXT

THE RAPEUTICS

The preliminary results **indicate** how rare a condition ulcerative colitis **is**.

Word - *Wise*

- indicate = show √

WORD ORDER

- how + adjective + a/an + noun + verb = how + rare + a + condition + ulcerative colitis + is = ulcerative colitis is a very rare condition

notes

-

cross REFERENCES

- *W* 27.33.36.37.47.48.51.

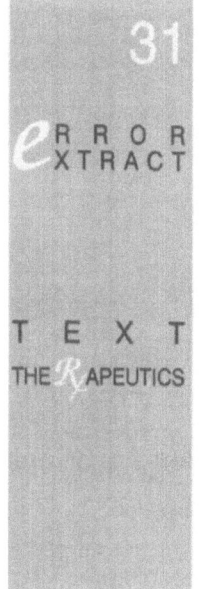

Eighteen patients with carcinoma of the pancreas had been studied preoperatively and 8 of these were studied on the 7th postoperative day after gastric bypass surgery.

Of the 18 patients with carcinoma of the pancreas who had been **evaluated** pre-operatively, 8 were **re-evaluated** on the 7th postoperative day **following** gastric bypass surgery.

prepositions

- out of the = of the > something that happens to one or several persons who are selected from a larger group = of the + 18 patients + 8 (were re-evaluated)

Word - _Wise_

- evaluate = assess; re-evaluate = re-assess

- following = after √

notes

-

-   •

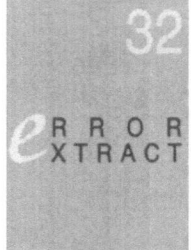

R R O R
XTRACT

However, patients who fail a first-line therapy do not have a favourable outlook.

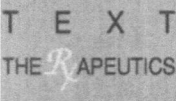

T E X T
THE RAPEUTICS

However, patients who fail a first-line therapy do not have a favourable **prognosis**.

However, **the outlook** for patients who fail a first-line therapy is not favourable.

insight

- *your* outlook = your general attitude towards a situation = perspective ≠ prognosis

- *the* outlook = how a situation will develop, improve or worsen = prognosis.

notes

-

c r o s s
REFERENCES

-   ●

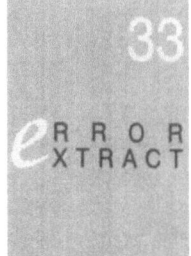

33

ERROR EXTRACT

In no patients any clinical improvement in the disease during and after treatment was observed.

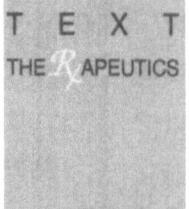

TEXT THERAPEUTICS

No clinical improvement in the disease was observed in **any of the patients either during or after treatment** .

In no patients was a clinical improvement in the disease **observed either during or after treatment**.

Grammar Glimpse

- no = not any = No clinical improvement was observed in any of the patients. = Clinical improvement was not observed in any of the patients.

insight

- broad negative (in no patients) at the beginning of a sentence (often for emphasis) + first part of two-part verb + subject + second part of two-part verb = in no patients + was + (a clinical) improvement (in the disease) + observed

WORD ORDER ⟶ ⟵

- subject + verb + modifier = (no clinical) improvement + was observed + either during or after treatment

c r o s s
REFERENCES

- *W* 27.30.36.37.47.48.51.   •

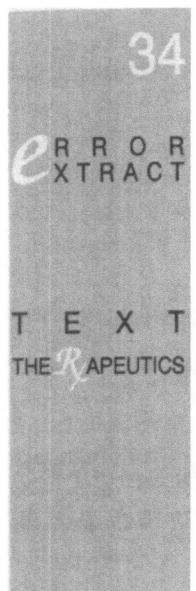

ERROR
EXTRACT

TEXT
THERAPEUTICS

As described before these patients had particular acute clinical features.

As has been described in the literature (by other authors), these patients had **particularly** acute clinical features.

verb ease
- present perfect tense > an action which began in the past and which continues in the present; although not directly stated, the underlying meaning of 'before' is: what has been written to date = to date + present perfect tense = as has been described in the literature (to date)

Specify
- state where: (as has been described) in the literature = as has been described before

Grammar Glimpse
- adverb + adjectives + noun = particularly + acute + clinical + features

cross REFERENCES
- v 4.8.11.12.17.23.24.25.26. • S 19.38.49. G 21.36. •

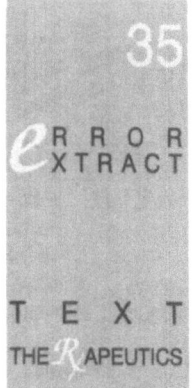

The seven-year results clearly indicate that when high-dose therapy is prescribed it is more effective than standard-dose therapy.

The seven-year results clearly indicate that **high-dose vs. standard-dose therapy is more effective**.

in *brief*

- high-dose vs. standard-dose therapy is more effective = when high-dose therapy is prescribed it is more effective than standard-dose therapy √

Word - *Wise*

- vs. = versus = as opposed to

notes

-

-

-

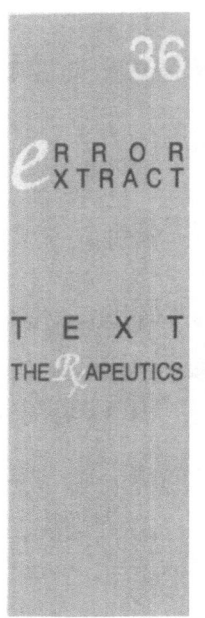

36

e R R O R
X T R A C T

T E X T
THE R APEUTICS

The strategy of giving high-dose therapy up front **is superior to** it's **use as salvage treat-ment** yielding a significant higher overall survival rate.

The high-dose therapy strategy, given up front, yields a significantly higher overall survival rate and is superior to **its** use as salvage treatment.

in *brief*

→
WORD ORDER
←

Grammar Glimpse

c r o s s
REFERENCES

- the high-dose therapy strategy, given up front = the strategy of giving high-dose therapy up front √

- subject + modifier + verb + object + con-junction [the subject is understood] + verb 'to be' + complement = (The high-dose therapy) strategy + given up front + yields + (a significantly higher overall survival) rate + and [this strategy] + is + superior to its use as salvage treatment

- adverb + adjectives + noun = (a) signifi-cantly + higher + overall + survival + rate

- its > relates to something previously mentioned ≠ it's = it is or it has (been)

- *W* 27.30.33.37.47.48.51. • *G* 21.34.   •

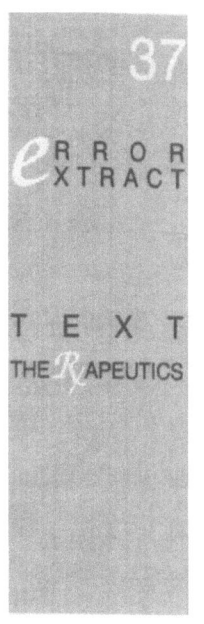

e R R O R
X T R A C T

Routinely with irradiation were treated 10 children who were in the first or second stage of the disease.

T E X T

THE *R* APEUTICS

Ten children who were in the first or second stage of the disease were **routinely** treated **with irradiation**.

Word Order

- subject + modifier + verb + modifier = ten children + who were in the first or second stage of the disease + were (routinely) treated + with irradiation.

- adverbs of frequency are usually placed between two-part verbs = were + routinely + treated

notes

-

c r o s s
REFERENCES

- *W* 27.30.33.36.47.48.51. • 8.10.25. •

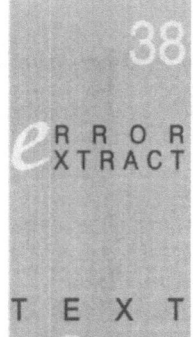

38

Toxicity is absent **and treatment can be** performed outpatiently.

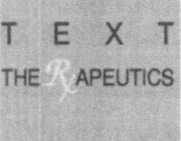

T E X T

THE *R* APEUTICS

Because of toxicity absence, treatment can be **administered on an out-patient basis**.

Specify	• state the reason why = because of + toxicity absence
Word - *Wise*	• administer = give = dispense = administer treatment
	• perform = carry out = e.g. perform surgery
	• on an out-patient basis ≠ outpatiently: 'outpatient' cannot be used as an adverb
notes	•

c r o s s
REFERENCES   • S 19.34.49.   •

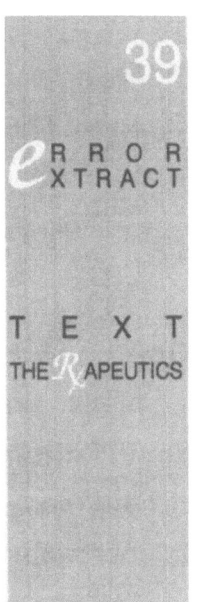

ERROR EXTRACT

It thus becomes possible to make retro-spective studies relating the proliferative activity to the clinical outcome.

TEXT

THE RAPEUTICS

It thus becomes possible **to do** retrospective studies relating the proliferative activity to the clinical outcome.

insight

- to do > an activity which involves the study of a subject = studies, research, a research paper, an abstract

- to do > laboratory work, your best

- to make > an activity related to speech = a speech, a comment, a point, a suggestion, enquiries

- to make > a change, alterations, an offer, a decision, a sound, a choice, a visit, a trip, a mistake, a note, a rule, a plan, sense

cross
REFERENCES

- •

•

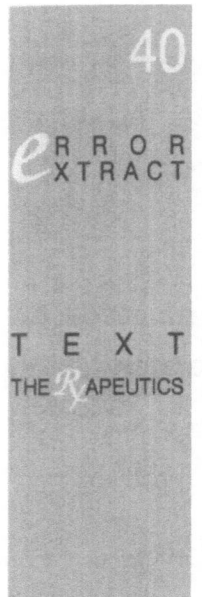

Moreover, the re-evaluation after two-thirds of first-line treatment plays an important role to identify as soon as possible the patient subset who require a modification of the chemotherapeutic approach.

Moreover, the re-evaluation **following** two-thirds of first-line treatment plays an important role **in the timely identification** of the patient subset **that requires** a modification of the chemotherapeutic approach.

Word - *Wise*

- following = after √

- timely = at the right time resulting in the prevention of problems or difficulties ≠ as soon as possible √

prepositions

- play a role in + noun = plays a role in (the timely) + identification; play a role in + 'ing' + noun = plays a role in + identifying + (the patient) subset

*G*rammar *G*limpse

- that > persons or things = the subset that; the patients that; who > persons = the patients who

- singular noun + singular verb = the (patient) subset + requires

c r o s s
REFERENCES

- *G* 27.50.   •

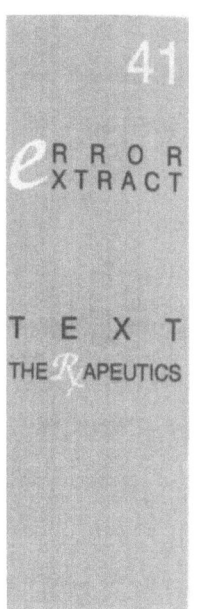

The merits of transplantation **for each particular patient** was evaluated with the ratio of probability of survival.

T E X T

THE *R* APEUTICS

Transplantation merits for each particular patient **were evaluated by means of the survival probability ratio**.

in *brief*

- transplantation merits = the merits of transplantation √

- the survival probability ratio = the ratio of probability of survival √

prepositions

- by means of > using a certain method or process to do or accomplish something: e.g. The merits were evaluated by means of the survival probability ratio. = The survival probability ratio was used to evaluate the merits.

Grammar Glimpse

- plural subject + plural verb = transplantation merits + were evaluated

c r o s s
REFERENCE

- *G* 7. •

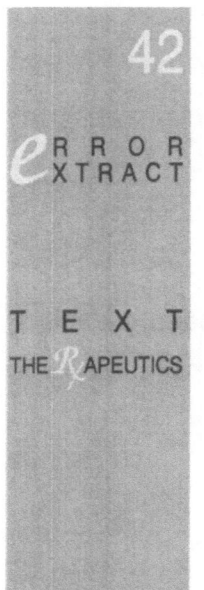

42

ERROR EXTRACT

This regimen is active and well-tolerated in aged patients but probably not enough active in younger patients.

TEXT

THE RAPEUTICS

Although in **elderly** patients this regimen is active and well-tolerated, in younger patients it is probably not **active enough**.

insight
- although + statement + surprising or unexpected second statement = although + it is an active and well-tolerated regimen in the elderly, + [unexpectedly] in younger patients it is not active enough

Word - *Wise*
- elderly = a polite reference to old people = old

- aged = very old

Grammar Glimpse
- adjective + enough + infinitive = (not) active + enough + to produce (the same results in younger patients)

cross REFERENCES
- •

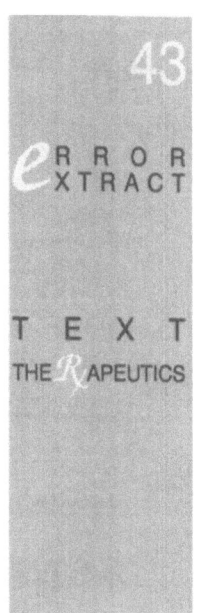

43

eR R O R
XT R A C T

All patients didn't have endocrine disease, their glucose levels were normal.

T E X T

THE **R**APEUTICS

In all patients glucose levels were normal and **all were without** endocrine disease. Glucose levels were normal in all patients and **none had** endocrine disease.

A V Ø I D

- contractions should not be used in professional publications: did not = didn't √

prepositions

- without = not to have something = without + noun = without (endocrine) disease

Grammar Glimpse

- all + affirmative statement = glucose levels were normal in all patients; all were without endocrine disease

- none + affirmative statement = none had endocrine disease

notes

-

c r o s s
REFERENCES

-

-

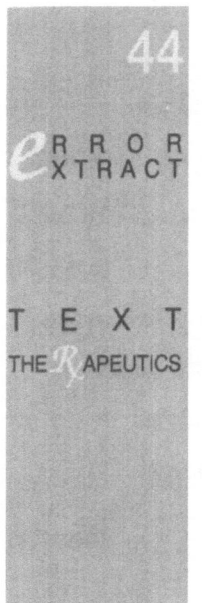

44

*e*R R O R
XTRACT

T E X T

THE R APEUTICS

The localisation of this receptor is not known and likely to be in the stomach.

The localisation of this receptor is **unknown but it** is likely to be in the stomach.

Word - *Wise*

• unknown = not known √

insight

• but > often follows a negative statement (or a statement negative in meaning) to introduce a second statement which is in reality (or most probably) the case = The localisation is unknown + but + it is likely to be in the stomach = We do not know where this receptor is located, but in all probability, it is in the stomach.

Grammar Glimpse

• two main clauses = subject + verb + conjunction + subject + verb = the localisation + is (unknown) + but + it + is (likely to be in the stomach)

c r o s s
REFERENCES

•   •

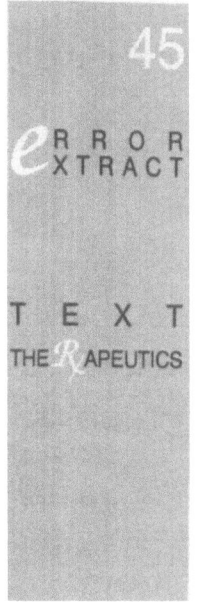

45

ERROR
EXTRACT

It is noted that in 7 cases more than twice biopsies were necessary in order to reach the diagnosis.

TEXT
THERAPEUTICS

It is notable (It has been noted) that in 7 cases more than **two** biopsies were necessary in order to reach the diagnosis.

Word - *Wise*

- noted = famous, renowned: e.g. He/she is a noted physician in the field of internal medicine.

- notable = noteworthy = worthy of note = it is notable

- it is noted = it is written = it is recorded = e.g. Confirmatory trials have been noted in the literature.

Grammar Glimpse

- plural number + plural noun = (more than) two + biopsies

- twice = adverb: verb + object + adverb = (we) repeated + (the) biopsies + twice

cross
REFERENCE

- G 20

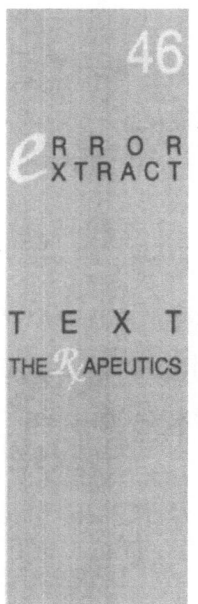

eR R O R
X T R A C T

This our early experience by the little number of treated cases has indicated lowest toxicity levels in all patients.

T E X T

THE *R* APEUTICS

Even though the number of treated cases was few, our early experience has indicated **low** toxicity levels in all patients.

insight

- even though = although + statement + second rather unexpected statement = even though + the number of treated cases was few + early experience has indicated low toxicity levels [and this is an unexpected result]

*G*rammar
Glimpse

- few + count nouns = e.g. few patients

- little + uncount nouns = e.g. little patience

- low = adjective = low toxicity levels

- lowest = superlative adjective > comparison of more than two persons, groups or objects: e.g. The toxicity levels were the lowest (of all) in group C.

c r o s s
REFERENCES

•   •

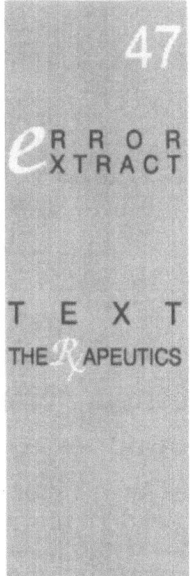

47

ERROR
EXTRACT

TEXT
THE RAPEUTICS

In this study we want to accentuate the priority of this method because only fewer complications are present which can be treated successfully.

Our aim in this study is to accentuate **the priority given to this method** because of the **fewer associated complications** which can be treated successfully.

Word - *Wise*

- our aim is = our objective is = we want to√

prepositions

- to give priority to + something = priority is given to + something = priority is given to + this method

WORD ORDER

- verb + object + modifier = accentuate + the priority + given to this method

in *brief*

- fewer associated complications = fewer complications are present √

notes

-

cross
REFERENCES

- *W* 27.30.33.36.37.48.51.

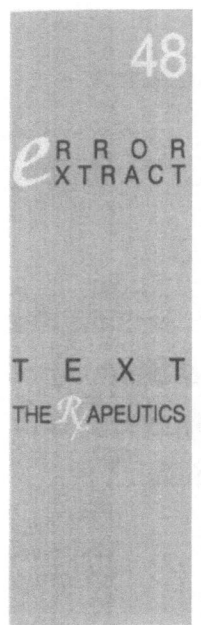

eR R O R
X T R A C T

Five groups of patients were observed with increased risks of poor response and of short rates of survival which allows us to identified **three prognostic groups with clear differences** in the duration of remission and in the duration of survival.

T E X T
THE *R*APEUTICS

Five groups of patients with **increased poor-response risks and short survival rates** were observed; **this allowed us to identify** three prognostic groups with clear differences **in both remission and survival duration**.

WORD ORDER

- subject + modifier + verb = five groups of patients + with increased poor-response risks and short survival rates + were observed

in *brief*

- increased poor-response risks and short survival rates = increased risks of poor response and of short survival rates √

- differences in both remission and survival duration = differences in the duration of remission and in the duration of survival √

verb ease

- allow + somebody + to do something = allowed + us + to identify

c r o s s
REFERENCES

- *W* 27.30.33.36.37.47.51. • v 1.3.6. •

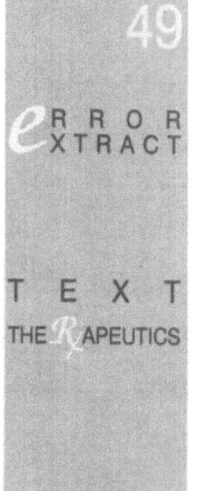

49

*e*RROR
XTRACT

The data are too preliminary to draw firm conclusions out of the feasibility of this protocol.

T E X T

THE ℞APEUTICS

As (since, because) the data are too preliminary, firm conclusions **regarding** the feasibility of this protocol **cannot be drawn**. **As (since, because)** the data are too preliminary, **we cannot draw** firm conclusions **regarding** the feasibility of this protocol.

Specify

- state why: as = since = because = as + the data are too preliminary

prepositions

- out of = outside of = away from: e.g. All of the pediatric unit staff are out of town at a medical congress.

- regarding = related to = regarding the feasibility

*G*rammar *G*limpse

- passive voice > the subject is often not mentioned = firm conclusions cannot be drawn (by us)

- active voice > the subject is mentioned = we cannot draw firm conclusions

c r o s s
REFERENCES

- S 19.34.38 • *G* 50. •

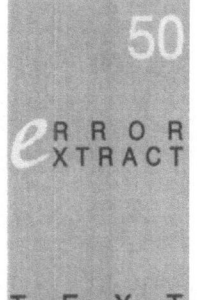

50

eR R O R
XT R A C T

Tissue material of the lymphomas were examined with **molecular genetic methods** confirming the original diagnosis.

T E X T
THE ℞APEUTICS

The lymphoma tissue material was examined by molecular genetic methods **and the original diagnosis was confirmed**.

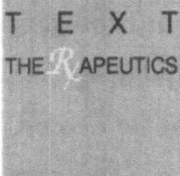

in *brief*
- the lymphoma tissue material = tissue material of the lymphomas √

Grammar Glimpse
- singular subject + singular verb = tissue material + was examined

verb ease
- smooth sentence structure > use two passive voice clauses in the same sentence = the material was examined and the original diagnosis was confirmed

prepositions
- by = by means of = using (particular methods or processes) = by molecular genetic methods

c r o s s
REFERENCES
- G 27.40. • v 49.   •

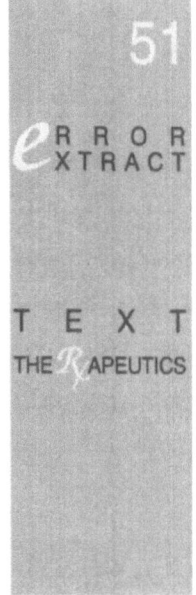

It is also noteworthy that the well-known prognostic parameters at diagnosis which identify patients not probably to be cured by conventional chemotherapy, are also associated with a poor outcome following more aggressive therapeutical procedures.

It is also noteworthy that the well-known prognostic parameters, **which at diagnosis identify patients who will probably not be cured** by conventional chemotherapy, are also associated with a poor outcome following more aggressive therapeutical procedures.

WORD ORDER

- subject + modifier clause + modifier clause + verb 'to be' + complement = (It is also noteworthy that) (the well-known prognostic) parameters + which at diagnosis identify patients + who will probably not be cured by conventional chemotherapy + are + also associated with a poor outcome following more aggressive therapeutical procedures

verb ease

- simple future tense > probability or certainty about a future action = (patients who) will probably not be cured by conventional chemotherapy = conventional chemotherapy will probably not cure these patients

c r o s s
REFERENCES

- *W* 27.30.33.36.37.47.48. •

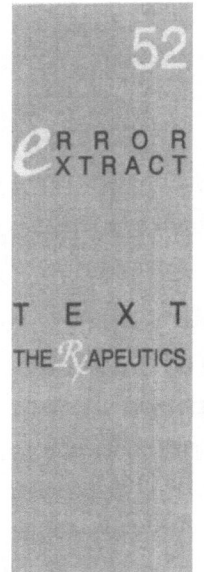

These results made it possible to have a distribution of 8 groups and a classification algorithm which determines survival probability.

These results made it possible **to identify** an **eight-group distribution** and **to establish** a classification algorithm which determines survival probability.

- to identify = to specify = to recognize = to identify an eight-group distribution

- to establish = to set up = to create = to establish a classification algorithm

- an eight-group distribution = a distribution of eight groups √

-

-

-

The following examples demonstrate some word order possibilities. S = subject, V = verb, O = object, M = modifier (adjective, adverb, phrase, clause).

- The scientist + expressed + his opinion.

  S + V + O

- The eminent + scientist + has stated + his opinion.

  M → S + V + O

- The noted + scientist + has + frequently + expressed + his opinion.

  M → S + auxiliary ← M → V + O

- The renowned + scientist + has + clearly + stated + his opinion + regarding the effectiveness + of this protocol.

  M → S + auxiliary ← M → V + O ← M ← M

- The distinguished + scientist + whose opinions are highly respected, + expressed + his views + related to the effectiveness + of this protocol.

  M → S ← M + V + O ← M ← M

Word
Order:
from the
Simple
to the
Complex

· A study + was initiated. (by us)

S + V

· We + initiated + a study.

S + V + O

· We + initiated + a pilot + study + in 1999.

S + V + M → O + [VM ←]

· [In 1999] + a multi-institutional + study + was initiated.

[VM→] + M → S + V

· A randomised + multi-centre + study + based on clinical stratification + was begun + in 1999.

M + M → S ← M + V ← M

· A co-operative + study + evaluating the therapeutic value of this treatment + was initiated + in 1999.

M → S ← M + V ← M

· [In order to evaluate the therapeutic value of this intensive treatment] + we + initiated + a pilot + study + based on clinical strati-fication.

[VM →] + S + V + M → O ← M

Useful Usage

CLINICAL +

- aggressiveness
- arena
- benefit
- criteria
- data
- deterioration
- effectiveness
- feature
- judgment
- picture
- remission
- significance

- clinical
- insufficient
- pertinent
- scant
- sparse
- sufficient

+ DATA

DIAGNOSTIC +

- approach
- criteria
- efficacy
- guideline
- process
- tool
- value

- aggressive
- bulky
- degenerative
- end-stage
- invasive
- multi-causal
- multifactorial
- protean
- recurrent
- relentless

+ DISEASE

Useful Usage

GENETIC +

compatibility
disparity
engineering
identity
lesions
machinery
marker
pathways

PROGNOSTIC +

impact
index
marker
model
parameter
significance

conditioning
curative
induction
low-dose
optimal
salvage
suboptimal
tailored
time-honoured

+ REGIMEN

THERAPEUTIC +

alternative
decision
implication
option
outcome
scheme
window

Useful Usage

ablative   + THERAPY
adjuvant
beneficial
combination
consolidation
curative
first-line
front-line
induction
intensification
maintenance
optimal
oriented
palliative
salvage
single-agent

case-control   + TRIAL
clinicopathologic
cohort
dose-ranging
double-blind
multi-institutional
parallel
pharmacodynamic
pilot
placebo-controlled
preliminary
randomised
retrospective
three-arm

As + SHOWN	= As + SYNONYM
	demonstrated
	displayed
	established
	exhibited
	highlighted
	indicated
	is evident
	observed
	pointed out
	presented
	projected
	set out
	specified
	substantiated

- … as shown **in** Table 1

- … as Table 1 demonstrates

- … as displayed **in** Figure 3

- … as Figure 3 indicates

- … as has been observed **in** the literature

- … as the literature has substantiated

- … as has been specified **by** other authors

- … as other authors have established

- … as is displayed **on** slide 4

- … as slide 4 highlights

A–Ω

An English Lexicon

The richness of the Greek language will improve your English vocabulary as well as enhance your research document and further elevate its level of professional excellence. What follows is a short English lexicon of words with Greek etymological roots.

- ACME: highest point of achievement or excellence

    ... the acme of perfection in health care

- ANTAGONIST: adversary

    ... an antagonist drug which acted in opposition to another prescribed therapy

- CATALOGUE: a list; to list

    ... to catalogue carcinogens

    ... we catalogued 104 cases

- CHARACTERISE: portray particular traits or features

    ... to characterise the disorder

- CRITERIA: standards by which to judge something

    ... the inclusion criteria of the trial

- CRITIQUE: a critical review; to critically review

    ... the process of critiquing the data

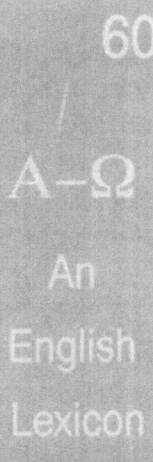

- DECADE: group of ten; ten years

  ... a decade of research

- DILEMMA: a situation involving a choice between difficult alternatives

  ... an aggressive vs. conventional patient management dilemma

- DRAMATIC: forceful, exciting

  ... dramatically different mutative capabilities

- DYNAMIC: active, energetic

  ... dynamic advances in oncological research

- EMPHASIS: importance; special attention

  ... the emphasis has shifted

- EMPIRICAL: based on observation and experience

  ... empirical treatment guidelines

  ... an empirical 3-6 month trial

- EPISODE: event or series of events

  ... an episode of pneumonia

- ETIOLOGY: study of causes

  ... as a consequence of etiologic factors

  ... the etiologically important role of

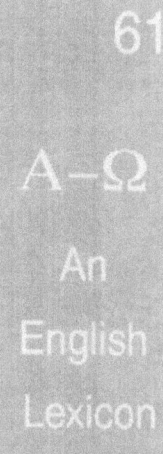

- GALAXY: a brilliant array

  … a galaxy of renowned scientists participated at the congress

  … a galaxy of medical talent

- GIGANTIC: enormous

  … gigantic steps forward in molecular biology

  … a gigantic achievement

- HELICAL: spiral

  … double helical DNA

- HERCULEAN: calling for courage and strength; difficult

  … a Herculean task in scientific research

- HOMOGENEOUS: composed of like parts

  … the stratification of cases into more homogeneous groups

- HYPOTHESIS: assumption, supposition

  … a working hypothesis

  … the hypothetical background of the experiment

- IDIOPATHIC: indicates unknown or uncertain cause

  … a case of idiopathic disease

- LETHARGIC: inactive, sluggish

  ... a lethargic clinical condition

  ... a lethargic patient

- LOGISTICS: related to organising something complicated

  ... the logistics involved in moving the patients to the new hospital wing

- MYRIAD: a large number, innumerable

  ... a myriad of animal studies

- OCTOGENARIAN: a person whose age is in the eighties

  ... a trial limited to octogenarians

- PLETHORA: overabundance, excess

  ... produces a plethora of antibodies

- PROTOCOL: a system of rules related to the correct way to proceed

  ... candidates for investigational protocols

  ... in the setting of protocol-based research

- PYROTECHNIC: brilliant, dazzling

  ... pyrotechnic surgical skills

- STRATA: section, level or division

  ... controls in both risk strata

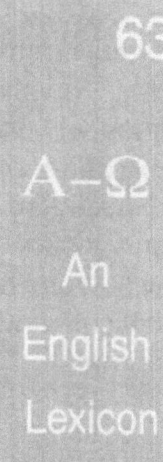

- STRATEGY: skill in managing or planning

  … a strategy to target resistant cells

  … a strategy of combined modalities

- SYMPTOMATIC: indicating active disease

  … before the development of the sympto-matic phase of the disease

- SYNCHRONOUS: occurring at the same time

  … synchronous worldwide trials

- SYNERGISM: simultaneous action of separate agents acting together and producing a greater total effect

  … synergistic action

- THEORETICAL: supposed to be true or to exist as stated; based on principles related to a particular subject

  … administration of this therapy is theo-retically sound

- TYPIFY: exemplify

  … a syndrome typified by abdominal distention

- ZEAL: intensive enthusiasm

  … scientific zeal

  … zealous endeavours to create a thera-peutic model

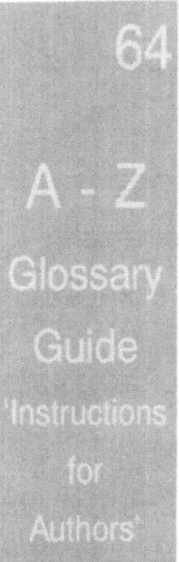

The 'instructions for authors' vary from medical journal to medical journal. Strictly adhering to the journal's guidelines will, in the long run, expedite the publication of your paper, once it is has been accepted. This glossary guide of terms and instructions (written in *italics*) will assist you in understanding the sometimes difficult and diverse terminology utilized by journals.

ABBREVIATIONS

- *...words or phrases for which abbreviations will be used should be spelt out first both in the abstract and in the text; the abbreviation follows in parenthesis...*

   > e.g. atrial fibrillation (AF), could not test (CNT), cytomegalovirus (CMV), long-chain fatty acid (LCFA); once the meaning is written in full first, the abbreviation may be used throughout the abstract and text

- *...do not use non-standard abbreviations in the abstract...*

   > approved abbreviations may be used; e.g. IgA = immunoglobulin A, IU = international unit, kg = kilogram, min = minute, NS = not significant; check the journal's list of standard abbreviations

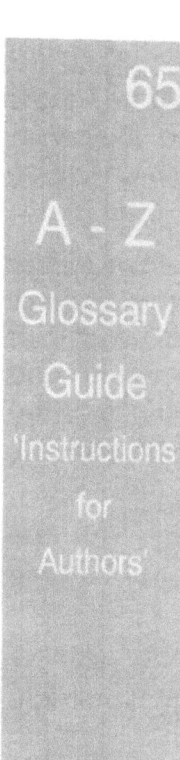

- *...do not use abbreviations in the title or abstract...*

  > spell out all words both in the title and abstract

- *...all abbreviations used in the paper must be listed below the key words...*

  > note every abbreviation in the paper under the key words (see KEY WORDS)

ABSTRACT (standard)

> abstract = summary; there are no sub-headings (see below)

ABSTRACT (structured)

> the abstract is divided into subheadings which usually include: objective, materials and methods, results, conclusions; other subheadings may include: background, study design, participants, interventions

AUTHOR(S)

> first, main, principal, senior author = the first author listed on an article

> author in charge of correspondence = the author who receives and replies to all correspondence from the journal

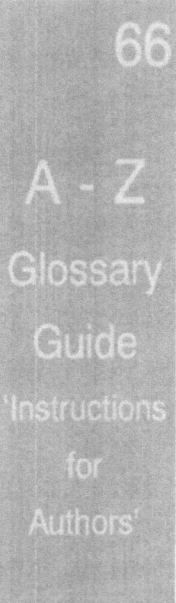

- *...the number of authors should be limited to six; if more authors are listed, the senior author must justify the inclusion of all authors...*

> specify the contributions of each author in the cover letter; e.g. who was responsible for: the first concept and design of the study, the data interpretation and analysis, the writing of the paper and the critical revision of the intellectual content

- *...the authors' names may not be appended after the manuscript has been submitted...*

> no additional authors' names may be added (e.g. at the revision stage) after you have sent in your paper

CONFLICT OF INTEREST

- *...in the cover letter, authors should disclose any financial arrangement they may have with a company whose product was used in the study, or with a competing company; such information may be printed at the end of the manuscript if it is accepted for publication...*

> the statement you make may be printed at the end of the published paper: e.g. 'This research was supported by ... whose product ... was used in this study.'

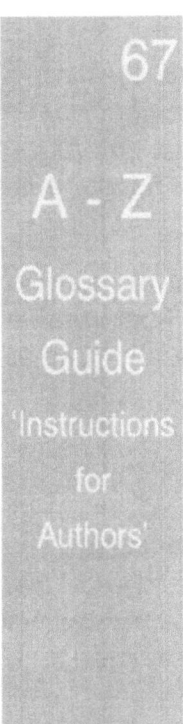
or, 'This research was supported by ... whose product ... is competitive to the product used in this study.'

COPYRIGHT TRANSFER

• *...the copyright transfer agreement (CTA) must be signed in original ink; the CTA is published in every issue of the journal and it may be photocopied...*

> the CTA may be photocopied from the journal but the photocopy must then contain the original signature of each author

COVER LETTER

> cover letter = transmittal letter = the letter which is sent to the journal along with your manuscript; it is signed either by all authors or the main author, or by the author in charge of correspondence

• *...the cover letter must state that the work has not been previously published and that it is not being considered for publication elsewhere...*

> e.g. 'We confirm that this manuscript has not been previously published and that it is not being simultaneously considered for publication elsewhere.'

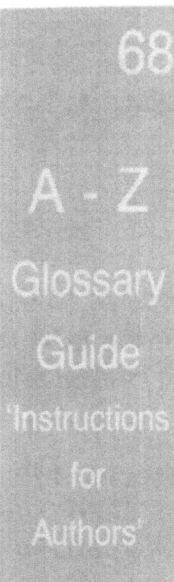
• *...the transmittal letter must include a statement confirming that all authors have read and approved the final version of the manuscript and concur with its submission...*

> e.g. 'This is to confirm that all authors have read and approved the final version of the manuscript and that we all agree to its submission.'

DISK (ELECTRONIC) SUBMISSION

• *...the label on the disk should include the name of the journal, the title of the article, the senior author's name, the number of files, hardware, software and version...*

> sample disk label:

Journal	*name of journal*
Manuscript title	*title of article*
Author(s)	main author, + et al.
No. of files	e.g. one;
	for more than one file
	note the content of
	each:
	e.g. two: text + tables
Hardware	e.g. Macintosh or PC
Software	computer program
	+ version number

FIGURES/LEGENDS

> figures may include illustrations such as: diagrams, flow charts, line drawings, graphs and photographs

> legends should sufficiently explain the data in the figure and they should not be printed on the figure themselves; what you see below the figures in published articles are the legends

• *...legends should be in consecutive order on a separate page...*

> the legends are printed separately (see MANUSCRIPT SEQUENCE), in a list, as shown below:

Legends

e.g. Fig. 1. CT scan of the abdomen...

e.g. Fig. 2. Histological section of the...

• *...when arrows, letters or numbers are used to identify an area of the illustration, these must be explained in the legends...*

> e.g. Fig. 3. ...calcifications (arrow) in the lower area of the...

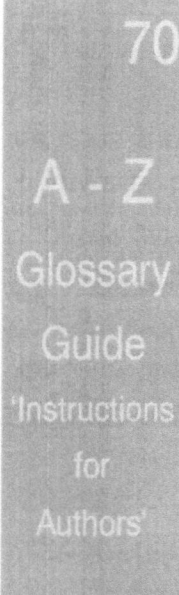

- *...for photomicrographs identify the method of staining and magnification data at the end of the legend...*

> photomicrograph = a photograph of a magnified image; e.g. Fig. 2. Histological section of the ... (H&E x 100). [i.e. hematoxylin and eosin stain x 100]

- *...affix an adhesive label to the back of each figure indicating the number and top of the figure, the senior author's name and the title of the manuscript...*

> make labels as shown and stick them to the back of the figures:

Fig. 1. Top ↑
Name of senior author
Title of manuscript

FOOTNOTES

- *...in tables, place explanatory matter and all non-standard abbreviations in footnotes...*

> use footnote symbols in this sequence in and at the end of the table: * † ‡ § || ¶

- *...footnotes should be avoided in the main body of the paper...*

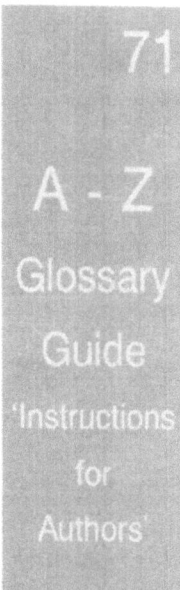

> footnotes may be used in tables but not in the text of the paper

HARD COPY

• *...disks must be accompanied by matching hard copy...*

> hard copy = on paper = the printed copy of your paper; the disk file(s) and the hard copy must be identical

HARD RETURNS

• *...use hard returns only at the ends of paragraphs, headings and subheadings...*

> let the text flow from one line to the next and use the computer's return key (↵) only at the end of the each paragraph, heading and subheading

HEADINGS

• *...main headings should be all caps (capital letters) and flush-left as indicated below...*

ABSTRACT

• *...main headings should be all caps and centered as shown...*

INTRODUCTION

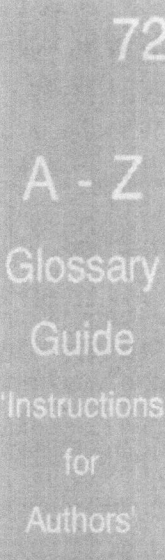

• ...*the first subheading should be caps plus lower case flush-left as shown...*

First Subheading

• ...*the second subheading should be cap plus lower case, indented and run-in text as in this example...*

Second subheading. Text follows here

INDEX MEDICUS

• ...*use the correct abbreviations for all journals as specified in the index medicus...*

> e.g. *Int J Card Imaging* = International Journal of Cardiac Imaging; journals whose titles are a single word, are not abbreviated: e.g. *Blood, Gut, Lancet*

INFORMED CONSENT

• ...*studies of human subjects must contain statements (in the Patients and Methods section) that the study was approved by the Institutional Review Board and that all subjects gave their informed consent...*

> e.g. 'This study was conducted with our Institutional Review Board's approval and all subjects gave their informed consent.'

A - Z
Glossary
Guide
'Instructions
for
Authors'

KEY WORDS

> key words are used for indexing purposes; choose words which will best describe your paper and list them alphabetically, (usually either on the title page or below the abstract)

LEGENDS (see FIGURES/LEGENDS)

MANUSCRIPT CATEGORIES

> check beforehand to verify that your work falls into one of the categories published by the journal and that it follows the guidelines and word count for that category; some manuscript categories are listed below

> brief report:
preliminary results of original research, concise descriptions of new findings

> case report:
unusual, new, innovative findings related to single cases

> editorial:
commentary on current issues or papers published in the same issue or on a recent finding published elsewhere; editorials are usually solicited by the editor

> letter to the editor:
comments on papers previously published in the journal and on current topics

> original (full) paper:
original research of major importance

> review article:
comprehensive overview and evaluation of the literature; often prior permission regarding the topic of the article is required from the editor

MANUSCRIPT SEQUENCE

> the manuscript is usually in this order:

1. Title page

2. Abstract or Summary

3. Text = Introduction + Patients (Materials) and Methods + Results + Discussion

4. Acknowledgements > if you wish to thank someone for his/her contribution to your paper; e.g. 'The authors wish to thank ... for his/her valuable contribution in analyzing the statistical data.'

5. References

6. Tables

7. Legends

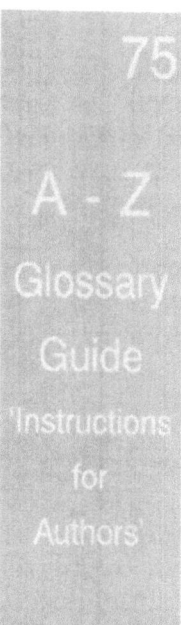

NUMBERS

- *...numbers one to nine should be spelled out except when used for percentages, degrees, dosages or when decimals are involved; for numbers above nine, numerals should be used...*

> except for percentages (5%), degrees (8°), dosages (1 g/m^2) and decimals (4.5), write out the numbers one to nine: e.g. eight patients; for numbers above nine, use the numeral: e.g. We enrolled 80 patients in the study.

OFFPRINTS (see REPRINTS)

PAGE CHARGES

- *...some of the publication costs are covered by a charge per printed page...*

> authors must pay the amount specified by the journal for each printed page of the article accepted for publication

- *...page charges beyond the first three printed pages are charged to the authors...*

> there are no page charges for printed pages 1-3; for printed pages 4 and above, the authors must pay a charge per page

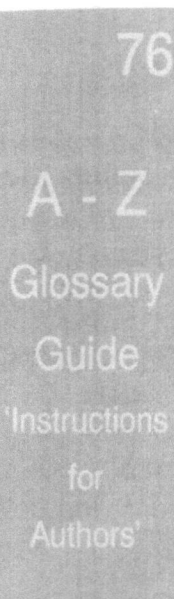

PAGE NUMBERS/FIRST AUTHOR'S NAME

- *...precede each page number (indicated in the upper right-hand corner of the page) with the surname of the first author...*

> e.g. Quinton - 5 = the first author's surname is Quinton and the page number is 5; use the 'header' dialog box on your word processing program

PAGE PROOFS

- *...authors will receive page proofs to correct and return within 48 hours of receipt; changes which involve the length of lines or pages will be made only at the authors' expense...*

> proofs = the pre-publication copy of your paper; these must be proof-read for minor corrections such as printer's or typographical errors; if major changes (alterations in the length of lines or pages) are made, the authors will be charged; journals require the corrected proofs within 48 hours in order for the article go to press in time

PARAGRAPHS

- *...indent the first line of each paragraph...*

> what you are reading now has the first line indented

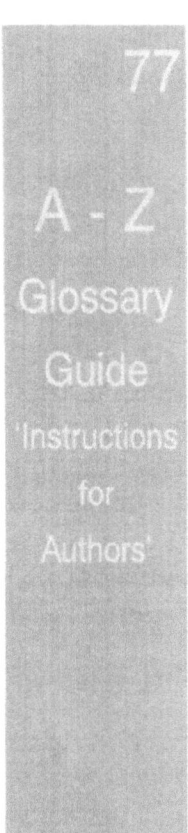

- *...do not right align...*

  > right align = right justify; what you are reading now is not right-aligned; notice that the right edge of this paragraph is jagged; the rest of this page is right-aligned/right-justified

- *...paragraph numbers should be indicated for all text pages...*

  1   Paragraph numbers tell you the number of the paragraph in relation to the rest of the text. This is paragraph 1.

  2   Refer to the instructions of your word processing program which will insert the paragraph numbers automatically.

  3   Every paragraph in the text must be numbered.

PERCENTAGES

- *...round off tenths of percents to whole numbers...*

  > 94.6% = 95%

- *...round off percentages to the nearest decimal point...*

  > 94.48% = 94.5%

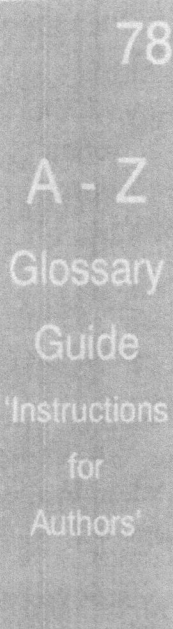

PERMISSIONS TO REPRODUCE TABLES OR ILLUSTRATIONS

- *...if the data used are from another published source, submit written permission from the copyright holder...*

> write to the Permissions Department of the journal or publisher and state: which data (table or illustration) you wish to use, the title of your article and the name of the journal to which it is being submitted for publication; e.g. 'We request permission to use ... for our article entitled, ... which is being submitted to ... for publication.'
> include the reply granting permission with your cover letter

- *...if adaptations have been made to a previously published table or illustration, permission to use an adapted version is required...*

> as above, specifying the adapted version (e.g. a previously published table + additional data)

- *...tables: acknowledgements of repro-duced material must be specified...*

> the source of the reproduced material should be cited below the table (not in the *Acknowledgements* section of your paper)

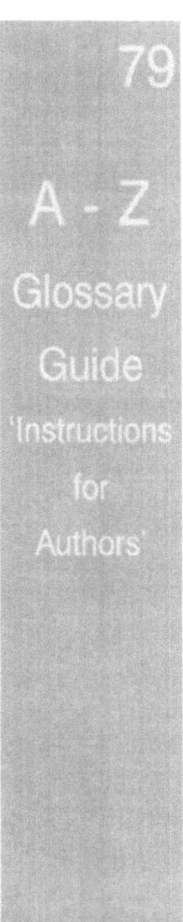

REFERENCE CATEGORIES

> follow the journal's formatting and punctuation for each category of reference; of the numerous types of references, the categories most often used are: standard journal article, personal author(s) of a book, conference proceedings, chapter in a book, volume with a supplement, issue with a supplement, editor(s), compiler(s) as author(s) and committee or corporate author; for a complete list of all reference categories, refer to: *Uniform requirements for manuscripts submitted to biomedical journals*. International Committee of Medical Journal Editors. *N Engl J Med* 1997;336:309-315.

REFERENCES

- *...indicate reference numbers in the text using parenthesis...*

  > (1), (2-4). = reference number(s) in parenthesis + punctuation

- *...indicate reference numbers in the text using square brackets...*

  > [5], [6-10]. = reference number(s) in square brackets + punctuation

- *...show reference numbers in the text using superscript...*

  > .[11-15] = punctuation + reference number(s) in superscript

- *...if there are six or more authors, list three + et al. ...*

  > six or more authors: omit all names except the first three authors + et al.

- *...use inclusive page numbers...*

  > e.g. 245-249

- *...if one page number only is given, specify whether the reference is an abstract or a letter...*

  > this is usually noted in square brackets after the title of the article; e.g. [abstract] or [letter]

- *...references must begin on a separate page in numerical order corresponding to the order of citation in the text...*

  > the reference section begins on a new page and references are listed by number in the order in which they appear in the text

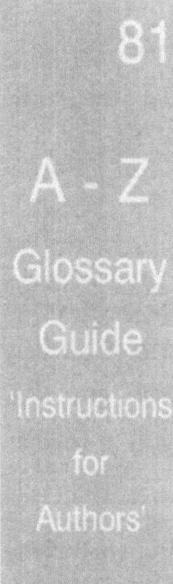

- *...references must be listed on a separate page in alphabetical order...*

> the reference section begins on a new page and the references are listed alphabetically

REPRINTS

> reprints = offprints = separately printed, single copies of your article

- *...the journal will provide reprints at a nominal fee...*

> nominal = minimal in comparison to the actual cost

- *...reprint orders accompanying the corrected proofs will be provided at a reduced price; the cost of reprints will be substantially higher after the article has gone to press...*

> if you order your reprints when you send in your corrected proofs, prior to publication, they will be much less expensive than if you order after the article is published

- *...order reprints in multiples of 100...*

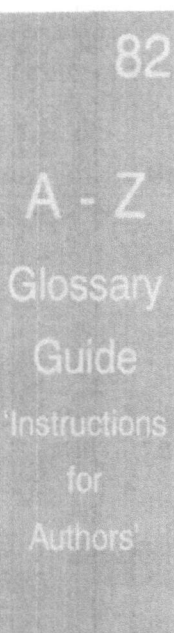
> the minimum order is 100 reprints; orders must be 100, 200, 300, etc. (i.e. you cannot order 150, 250, etc.)

REVIEWERS

• *...authors may submit the names of three reviewers (who are not on the Editorial Board of the Journal); supply their names, addresses, phone/fax numbers and e-mail addresses, in the cover letter...*

> you may suggest reviewers, provided they are not members of the Editorial Board of the journal; note their names and details as specified above, in the transmittal letter; e.g. 'We would like to suggest the following three reviewers: ...'

RUNNING HEAD

> running head = running title = short title = the shortened version of the actual title of your paper; the running head is what you see printed (usually at the top of every second page of the published paper); in the submitted version of your paper the running head is usually noted at the bottom of the title page

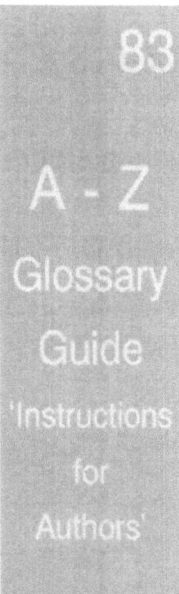

• *...the running head must not exceed 50 characters...*

> count both letters and spaces; the above instruction = 46 characters

SPELLING

• *...spelling may be British or American but must be consistent throughout...*

> use either British or American spelling but not both in the same document; e.g. British/American spelling: colour/color, tumour/tumor, haematology/hematology, anaemia/anemia, ischaemic/ischemic

> when writing for American or British journals, use the relevant spelling

> note: in some examples in this book, British spelling is used, in others, American spelling

SUMMARY (see ABSTRACT)

TABLES

• *...use a separate numbered page for each table...*

> each table should be on a single page on its own

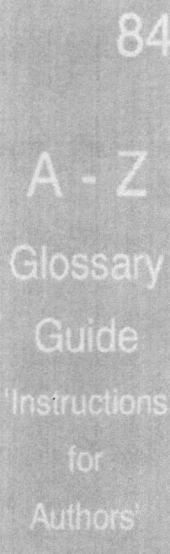

- *…do not use internal horizontal or vertical lines…*

  > use no lines whatsoever inside the table

- *…do not use internal horizontal or vertical rules…*

  > as above; use no lines inside the table

- *…use Arabic numbers…*

  > Table 1.

- *…use Roman numerals…*

  > Table II.

- *…save tables as a separate file as 'text only'…*

  > use the 'save as' option on your word processing program and select 'ASCII text' or 'text only' for the tables; the disk you submit should have a separate file for the tables

TITLE PAGE

- *…authors should be identified by their first names, middle initial(s) and surnames; do not include titles and academic degrees of authors…*

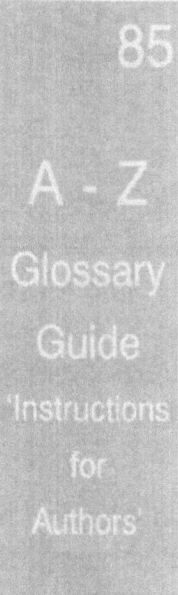

> omit title(s) such as professor, and academic degree(s) such as MD, PhD; e.g. Zachary S. Quinton

- *...authors should be identified by their first names, middle initial(s), surnames and highest academic degree...*

> e.g. Zachary S. Quinton, MD

- *...use superscript footnote numbers to indicate affiliations...*

> e.g. Zachary S. Quinton,[1] Benjamin L. Walker,[2] Sandra P. French,[3]...
[1] Department of ..., institution, city, country, [2] Department of ..., institution, city, country, [3] Department of ..., institution, city, country

- *...use superscript footnote letters to indicate affiliations...*

> e.g. Zachary S. Quinton,[a] Benjamin L. Walker,[b] Sandra P. French,[c]...
Department, institution, city and country as above, using letters

- *...use superscript footnote symbols to indicate affiliations...*

> e.g. Zachary S. Quinton,[*] Benjamin L. Walker,[†] Sandra P. French,[‡] ...
Department, institution, city and country, as above, using footnote symbols

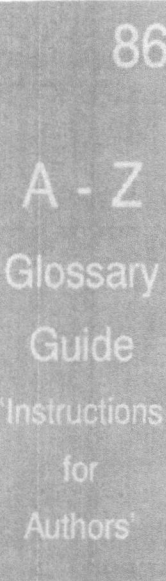

TRANSMITTAL LETTER (see COVER LETTER)

WELFARE OF ANIMALS

• *...all studies on animals must contain a statement (in the Materials and Methods section), that the care of the animals was in accordance with the institution's guidelines or some other internationally recognized guidelines for ethical animal research ...*

> e.g. 'The guidelines of our institution (or of ...) for the use, care and handling of animals for research were respected.'

WORD COUNT

• *...include the word count of the abstract after the key words at the bottom of the abstract page...*

> word count = the number of words in a given area of the text: e.g. abstract word count = 150; note this at the bottom of the abstract page; use the 'word count' facility on your word processing program

• *...include a word count of the text (excluding the abstract, references and tables) at the bottom of the title page...*

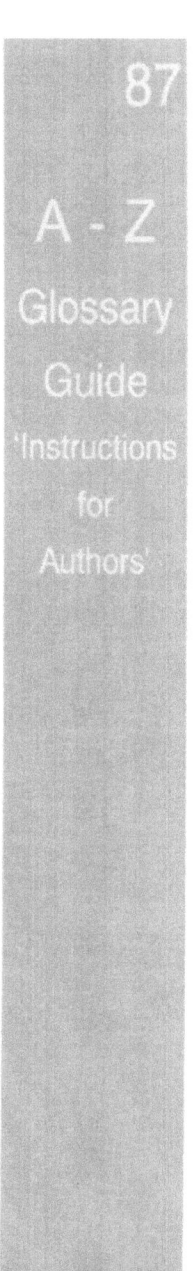

> note at the bottom of the title page: e.g. text word count = 2654; select the text in your paper starting at the *Introduction* and ending at the last word in the *Discussion* and use the 'word count' facility, as above

ZIP CODE

• *...provide the complete address including the zip code...*

> zip code = postal code = numbers and/ or letters which are part of an address: e.g. ON, N8A 3H1, Canada; Boston, MA 02116, USA; GR-116 35, Athens, Greece; FR-75004, Paris, France